No Bullshit Weight Loss

Thomas Ap Dewi

To all the unsuccessful dieters who would die young anyway.

CONTENTS

Introduction: It's your life - live it how *you* want

Losing weight is a necessity if you want to look good. Sure, it can help you to lead a longer and healthier life, but frankly, we don't care about that. Health and wellbeing is not a priority for us - slimming down your fat ass is.

With that in mind, a large proportion of the advice in this book is bad for you, hazardous to your health, and as any doctor will tell you, should not be considered as a long-term alternative to a fitness regime and healthy eating. Some of it is illegal.

That's the disclaimer out of the way. We are totally advocating that you adopt the advice contained herein as a lifestyle choice. Your life will be considerably shorter, but we promise you two things: You will be slimmer, and you will have more fun. And life's all about looking good and having fun. You may even become more productive, make friends and influence people. But we're not making any promises on that score.

We don't know what you look like. The only thing we know about you is that you think you're overweight, and you want to remedy that, with zero regard for your general wellbeing. We dig it. You could be a slightly plumpish lady in her twenties who has tried everything else, or you could be a thirty stone monster of a man, and you never stir from the couch as you have the beer fridge right next to you and you piss into the empty cans. It doesn't matter. Follow this lifestyle advice and you will half your body mass in no time at all.

There are a lot of diets out there which promise to make you thin in a couple of weeks or months, and while they may help you to shed a few pounds, the weight soon piles back on as soon as you give them up. And dieters do give them up. Because they're hard. Completely cutting out all sugar and fat? That's difficult. A regular exercise regimen? No-one has the time for that bullshit.

We won't be asking you to give up KFC or Nando's, and we won't be telling you to haul your fat ass out of bed at five in the morning to go for a run or compete in your own personal triathlon.

Healthy home cooking? Leave it for someone who cares about that kind of stuff. Join Weightwatchers. Whatever.

For the sake of balance, and so that you can make an informed choice, we'll be providing potential downsides along with our weight loss advice. This isn't meant to discourage you in any way, and frankly, it's just so that we don't end up being sued - kind of like those huge contra indication sheets you get along with oral contraceptives. Read it or not. Like everything else in your life, it's your choice.

There is very little willpower involved in any of the advice this book offers, however, perseverance and commitment is required - Don't give up! Buying this book is the first step towards a slimmer you!

Caffeinate up, bitches

You know who looks really good? All sexy and slim and really, really wide awake?

College students, that's who. And the reason for this is twofold. College students are young, or they tend to be, anyway. Young people have fast metabolisms, and what this means is that they can eat whatever the hell they want and stay skinny, just like you want to. Right?

Fats, proteins and fried foods all get broken down quickly and flushed out before they are used by the body to build up new tissue. While this means that fat doesn't pile on from all of the late night pizza and beer we all love so much, it also means that they don't pile on muscle as easily, and have to work harder than older people to gain muscle mass.

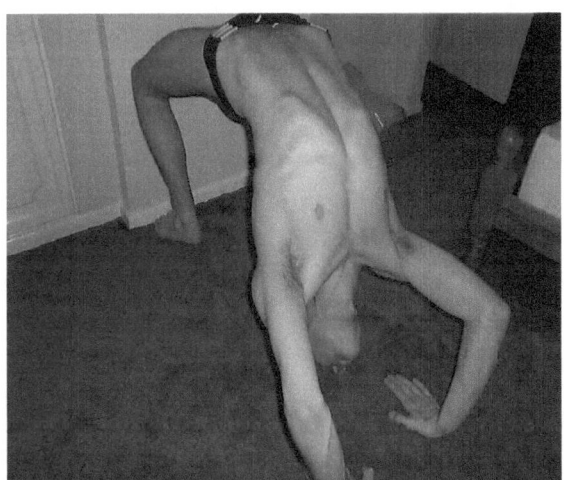

Figure 1: This guy

Yes, it is possible to find fat college students, but take it from us, you're looking at them at their slimmest. If you think they're fat now, wait until you see them 20 years down the line, they're at their slimmest and most beautiful, but if they follow the advice in this book, they can prevent that downward spiral too.

Another contributory factor to the general slimness of college students is that they have essays and assignments they leave to the last minute. On the night before deadline, students stay up all night ploughing away on a mixture of coffee and Red Bull (other energy drinks are available).

That's where it's at. Caffeine.

Caffeine has a massive and pronounced effect on weight loss. It stimulates the nervous system to send signals direct to the fat cells telling them to start breaking down fats; it also stimulates the production of adrenaline, which reinforces the message by pummelling the fat cells into submission.

The chemical can also increase the resting metabolic rate by between 3% and 30%, meaning that you can actually increase the amount of crap you eat and carry on losing weight.

The problem is that you're probably not a college student. The metabolic effect of caffeine is less pronounced in older people, and you're probably not looking at more than a 10% base increase in metabolic rate. But there's a simple answer here too. You need to consume huge quantities of caffeine on a regular basis.

Think of how much coffee a night-shift investment banker working 18 hour shifts drinks. Is that a lot of coffee? It's not enough.

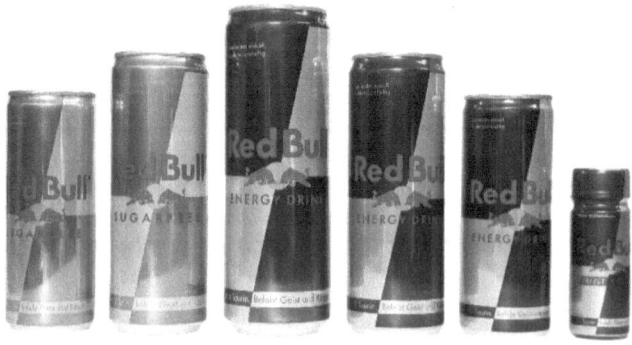

Figure 2 Not nearly enough

Double that amount of coffee and then throw a few caffeinated energy drinks down the hatch. Daily.

There's also the added bonus that coffee contains both Theobromine and Theophylline, closely related compounds with a similar stimulant effect, and chlorogenic Acid, which acts to slow the absorption of carbohydrates.

The downside:

Seriously, consuming coffee and energy drinks in the quantities we're advocating is going to mean that you don't get much sleep - there's another section on this, and it isn't necessarily a bad thing.

In addition, you're likely to suffer from restlessness, increased heart rate (at least it's working - right?), nausea, anxiety, sweating, dizziness, and vomiting.

In a worst case scenario, excessive caffeine consumption can cause cardiac arrest - also known as a heart attack - meaning that you may die.

Party like it's 1989

Remember how we said there would be no exercise involved in this book? Well, we were lying. Sort of.

What we want you to do here is pretend that it's 1989 again. You may have been there the first time round - we don't know. If you were, the chances are that you were in a hell of a lot better shape than you are now.

The late 1980s were glorious if you were involved in the right scene, and we're not referring to Michael Jackson glory years or to Madonna concerts either. We're referring to the underground rave scene.

Vast warehouse parties, stuffed to bursting point with thousands of sweaty bodies, dancing hard. All night. Literally from dusk till dawn.

Dancing is awesome. We see people doing in park or in dancercise groups where everyone bops gently in time with the instructor. Don't do that - it's bullshit. Also, don't buy the Wii fit dancing game because that's bullshit too.

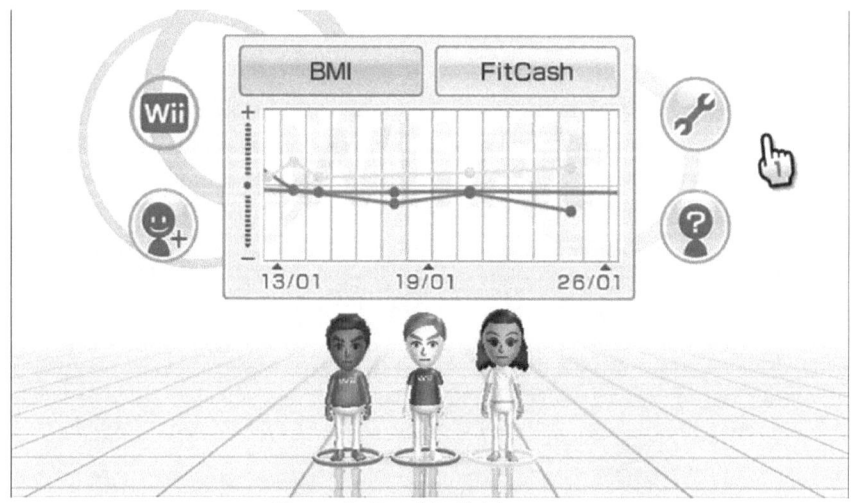

Figure 3: Total bullshit

Proper, hard dancing can burn as much as 800 calories an hour, and we're suggesting you pull a 12 hour shift here.

Yes you're right. There's no way in hell that you can dance that hard for that long. We know, no-one can.

Not without chemical assistance that is.

An integral part of the warehouse rave scene was the drug culture which accompanied it - without a bespoke blend of consumer pharmaceuticals, rave never would have existed. Normal people simply don't have the stamina to keep moving for that long.

While there was a great deal on offer, and there still is, we suggest that you stay away from heroin, and crack.

What you should be looking for are ecstasy and speed, also known as amphetamine. We'll look at speed first.

Speed is a stimulant. It keeps people awake, alert and full of energy. On speed, you can do literally anything for hours and end. You'll be able to dance, talk, walk, and just keep going. It doesn't matter that your body is essentially a flabby sack of butter, you will dance and get more exercise in one night than you have in the last twenty years combined.

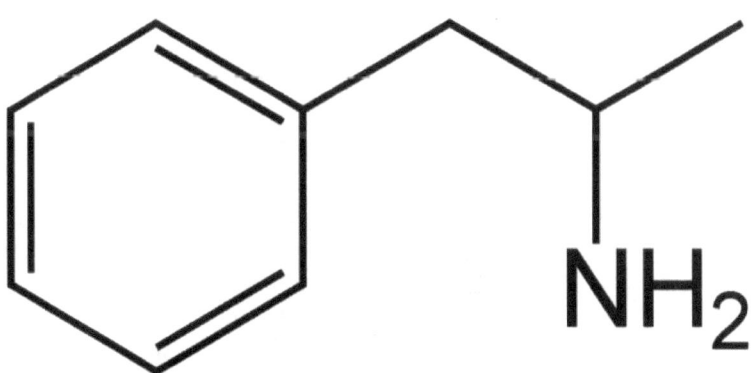

Figure 4: This guy

As an exra added bonus, speed also speeds up your heart - it's getting a double workout from the dancing and from the pills. Pretty natty, huh?

Ecstasy (or MDMA) will make you feel alive and in tune with your surroundings, as well as giving you energy. If you're a shy retiring wallflower, who tends to stay away from dance floors for risk of being ridiculed, you're going to need ecstasy to help you to get over that. Take MDMA and you're guaranteed to develop feelings of love and affection for the people you're with and for the strangers around you. Ecstasy will help you to get over your initial shyness, and move your comfort zone so far out that you'll be willing to give anything a go.

After 12 hours dancing on a mix of MDMA and amphetamine, we estimate that you will have burned around 13,000 calories.

Keep it up once per week - you'll love it and the weight will just fall off your body like it was never there (apart from some stretch marks maybe).

The downside:

Narcotics. Do you know where to get them? Probably not. Chances are that unless you know a reliable dealer, you're going to be busted by the law and the only exercise you'll be getting is repeatedly picking up the soap. You might also be beaten or killed if you're buying in the wrong part of town.

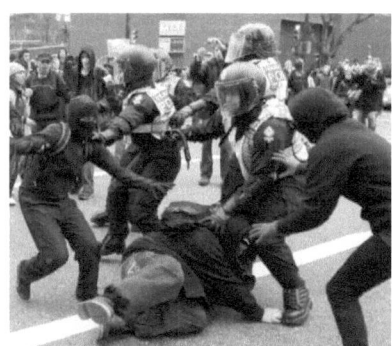

Figure 5: It could be you in this picture

Amphetamine can put a strain on your heart, and people have actually died of heart attacks after taking too much speed. Moderation is the key. You will also feel irritable during the comedown period

The effects of ecstasy wear off after three hours or so, and you might suddenly feel out of place and be tempted to take more. Whether you do or not is up to you, but bear in mind that short term side effects include feeling anxious or getting panic attacks. There aren't really any genuine health risks associated with ecstasy, however it is important to stay hydrated. Not too hydrated though - there's been at least one death where a girl died after drinking too much water while on ecstasy.

Commune with the spirits

Are you the kind of fatty who spends their evenings chilling out on the couch with the love of your life, watching Supernatural on Netflix, munching Pringles, and drinking red wine or beer?

Yeah. We thought so, but you need to can that shit right now and get with the programme. You can keep the Supernatural and the Pringles, but you urgently need to dump the red wine and the beer in favour of something a bit stronger. Like Vodka.

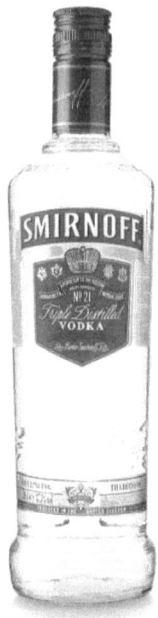

Figure 6: This. We like this.

The benefits of vodka are many and varied. Russians drink it all the time instead of water or coffee even. In Russia, beer is considered a soft drink. Russians don't drink soft drinks.

We know from research and personal experience that red wine is good for you - its stuffed with anti-oxidants and it's a vasodilator, meaning that it widens blood vessels - giving your heart a workout and making you horny. As part of a balanced diet, red wine is a good thing healthwise. But you're reading this to get slim, not to get healthy.

Red wine contains around 700 calories per bottle, while beer is packing in the region of 200 calories per pint. And they're calories you can do without.

On the other hand, vodka contains no carbohydrates or fats and has very few calories. That is exactly what you need.

Vodka also gets you very drunk, very quickly. At least, it gets us very drunk, very quickly. Your mileage may vary. If you're following the advice in this book, then by the early evening, you'll be an over caffeinated wreck. Without help, you won't be able to get to sleep at all, and you will, at some point need to sleep, especially if you have been out all night popping pills at an underground rave.

Substituting vodka for wine means that you need to drink it at the same rate. By our calculations, this means that you should be unconscious before the first Supernal episode has finished, so make sure that Netflix isn't queued to auto-play.

In addition to eschewing the wine and beer calories, it's also unlikely that you'll manage to reach the bottom of the Pringles tube as your coordination will start to deteriorate after a few glasses, and you'll be unconscious long before you reach the bottom of the bottle. More calories saved. Double bonus! Let's make that a quadruple bonus by giving you such a colossal hangover that even the thought of your customary fried grits breakfast has you running for the toilet to hurl the contents of your stomach against the porcelain. Not only have you dodged the breakfast calories, you've also managed to rid yourself of the Pringles calories from the night before.

Now go and make some coffee.

The downside:

If this is a nightly thing with you, you may start to develop the symptoms of alcoholism. These include, but are not limited to:

jitters, shakes, excess sweating, and eventually brain damage.

There is also the danger that you either stop going to work, or show up smelling of vomit and last night's vodka. People may not want to sit next to you.

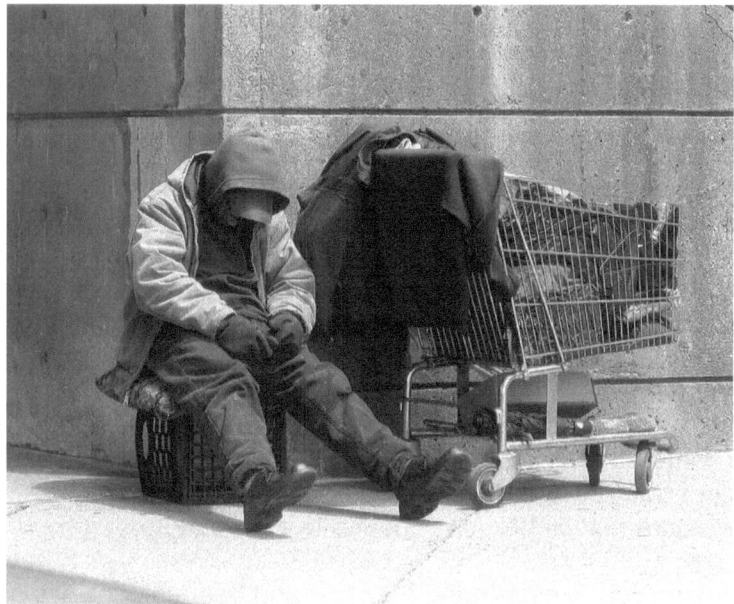

Figure 7: This could be you.

Smoking Thrills

Smoking is one of those areas where civilisation seems to have developed a sort of collective amnesia over the last couple of decades.

It's been known for around a century that cigarettes kill people - it's never been a secret, and yet, for some reason, cigarette companies are now trying to say that it's news to them, and being forced to pay out millions in compensation to the families of people who have been killed by smoking related diseases. We don't know why, and we don't care too much either.

For the longest time, tobacco companies targeted young housewives - a traditionally non-smoking segment of society with adverts claiming that taking up the habit would help them to stay slim and keep their husbands interested.

Why? Because it's the 100% God's honest truth. Cigarettes totally work as a means of both losing weight and keeping the weight off. And they work in oh so many different ways. If you're trying to lose weight and you don't smoke, you should totally take it up.

The most obvious contributing factor to smoking as a means of losing weight is that if you have a cigarette in your mouth, you can't put anything else in there. Makes sense, right? Well you probably can manage to slide a few Doritos past the nicotine stick, but the whole experience is unpleasant. You don't want that, trust us.

Aside from that slightly silly example, nicotine is a genuine, actual factual appetite suppressant. Simply having it in your bloodstream will make you less hungry because it affects the muscles in the walls of your stomach, causing a damping effect on any hunger pangs you may be having. Chain smoking keeps those nicotine levels sky high, and with an intake of four packets of Marlboro per 24 hour period, it's possible to go for days at a time without feeling even a little bit peckish.

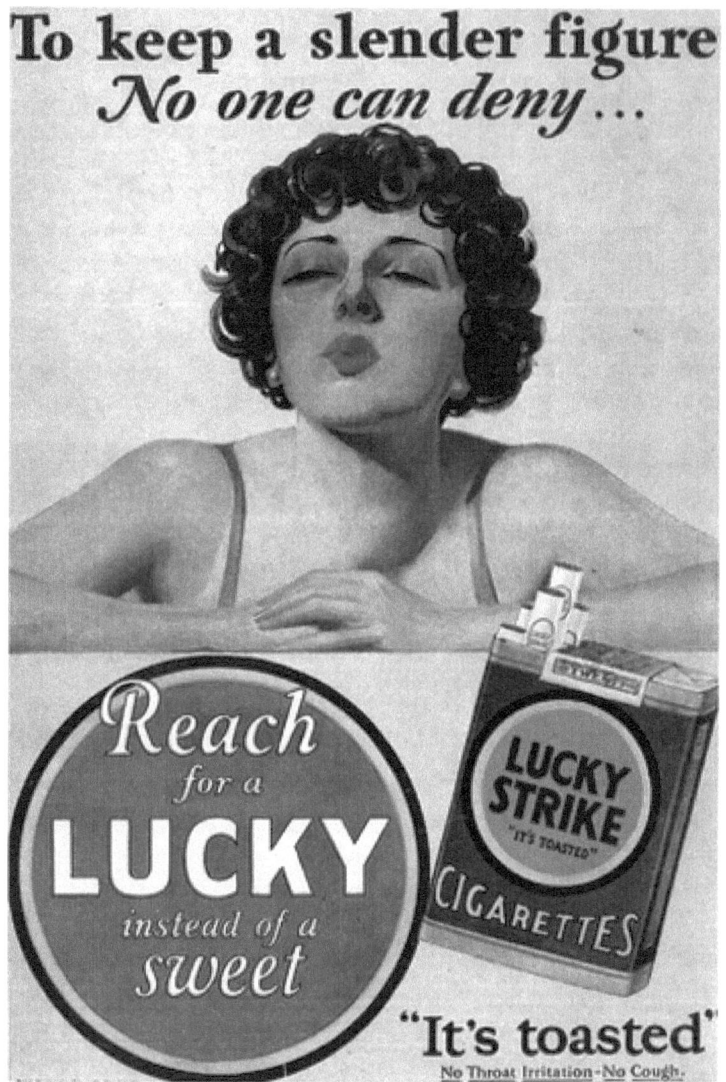

Figure 8: No-one is denying it, sweetheart.

Again, this isn't new knowledge, South Americans knew about the link between tobacco and weight loss well before Columbus set his booted feet on their sacred shores, and the first ships to bring the weed back to Europe had it figured out pretty quickly too.

The third way smoking helps you lose weight is that old favourite - it's a metabolism booster. The faster your metabolism, the less weight you put on and the easier it is to lose it. Combined with coffee, cigarettes can push your metabolism through the roof.

You're also likely to expend more calories while engaged in activity. We don't know why this is. It could be that your lungs are so deteriorated that it takes a whole lot more effort to even breathe, but whatever. Cigarettes work.

In the 1960s, cigarette manufacturers were set up directly against candy companies and ran parallel advertising campaigns, both promising short term energy and distraction, but with the nicotine pedallers promising boosts to mental agility and the overwhelming attraction of not becoming a lard-ass through habitual use over an extended period. They were right, too.

The downside:

Where to start?

Short term negative effects include a rapidly appearing 'smoker's cough,' and being forced to stand outside restaurants, bars, cafes, and your place of work.

You will smell. You might not notice it, but non-smokers will and they will get in your face about it. For some reason it's considered socially acceptable to be openly rude to and about smokers, so you're likely to become a magnet to obese puritans giving you shit about polluting their air.

The longer term effect is that your health will go to hell. Not immediately, but you're looking at chopping a couple of decades of your lifespan before succumbing to either heart disease or lung cancer.

This can be either a good thing or a bad thing depending on how you look at it. Yes, you die prematurely, but at least you don't live long enough to need 24 hour care because you can't remember your name and you've lost the ability to control your own bladder. As far as we're concerned, the jury is still out on that one.

Eat out and eat dirty

You should eat out once in a while. No - we don't mean the kind of eating out you're thinking of, although we're generally in favour of that too.

It's a little known fact that around 5% of all females in the western world are bulimic - this means that they deliberately make themselves sick so as to not put on weight from the food they've just eaten. The sad part is that it's generally girls who are underweight who do this. They don't need to lose weight, whereas you do.

We're not so irresponsible to suggest that you ram your fingers down the back of your throat to barf up your breakfast. There's no joy in that, and besides, it's an effort. We promised you no effort, and we're sticking by that.

No. We're fully in tune with your lifestyle and we want you to continue what you're doing - go a little further in fact.

We want you to start visiting the worst food joints you can find. Pop up fly by night vendors, who are just one step away from being closed down by the food standards agency.

Look for signs such as the chef having a piss in the alley behind the venue, or nests of rats just outside the doorways and around the bins. If you live in a town where there are no such establishments, then you may need to venture out at three in the morning or whenever the nightclubs start kicking out near where you live. There is bound to be an array of hot dog and hamburger vendors queued up near the taxi rank ready to serve the unwary with a healthy dose of food poisoning.

And that's what we're after.

If you're lucky, these mobile eateries with their unsanitary practices will have their onion vats swimming in a pool of bacteria such as salmonella or Escherichia coli (E. coli), or even viruses, such as the norovirus.

Once you have contracted one of these diseases, give it a couple of days to incubate, and you will completely lose your appetite and will to eat with no additional effort required. Not only that, but you will completely lose the contents of your stomach through both diarrhoea, and through vomiting, like those unfortunate bulimic girls mentioned above.

And just because your stomach is empty doesn't mean the weight loss benefits are over.

If you're lucky, your symptoms may persist for more than a week, meaning that every time you put something in your mouth, it instantly reappears before your body has had time to digest it.

Within a week, it's entirely feasible that you could have lost as much as 20 pounds. That's pretty impressive.

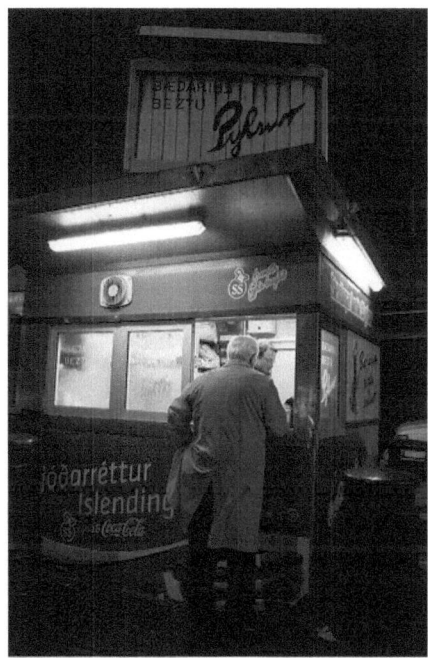

Figure 9: POtentially the answer to all of your weight loss problems

The downside:

You'll be ill and will probably have to take some time off work. If you've been following the 'party like it's 1989' step, the chances are that you're now unemployed, and if they haven't sacked you yet, this may be the last straw.

Being ill is unpleasant. Aside from the vomiting, if you deliberately contract food poisoning, you may also run a fever.

Long term use of this weight loss tip may result in stomach acid permanently damaging your teeth, and possibly even an ulcer if you're unlucky.

Snack Attack

Hey! You're hungry because your stomach is telling your brain that there's nothing in there, or that there's more space which needs filling up.

If you've taken up smoking, as recommended, these signals will be weaker and less frequent, but if you're still subject to the pangs, then you need to fill that gap. Like we said at the beginning, we're not asking for willpower anywhere in this book, so if your stomach is telling you it needs to be filled, then you can fill it.

What usually happens when you eat is that enzymes go to work as soon as food passes your lips. Amylase breaks down long carbohydrate chains into shorter sugars ready to be absorbed. When the food hits your stomach, chemicals get busy with it, breaking it down further and squishing it and squashing it before passing it on to the intestines where further absorption and mechanical action takes place. The bottom end of your intestine is the rectum and anus, and by the time what was food reaches there, all nutritional value should have been extracted. With us so far? Good.

What you should have gleaned from that teeny bit of science is that calories, fats and carbs are being extracted throughout the whole process, but you need to eat or your stomach will be screaming for more.

The trick is, to fill up your stomach, but with something from which no calorific or nutritional benefit can be extracted whatsoever. Something which takes up space, can pass through your gastro-intestinal tract, make your stomach feel full, and yet not make you put on weight. There's an added bonus if it can be chewed too.

"So, what is this wonder food?" I hear you ask.

Literally anything that isn't food and won't poison you, will do the trick. Paper is good, it will fill your stomach yet not be digested because humans can't break down the cellulose from which paper is made.

We particularly recommend toilet paper due to it's texture and how easily it disintegrates while still taking up space.

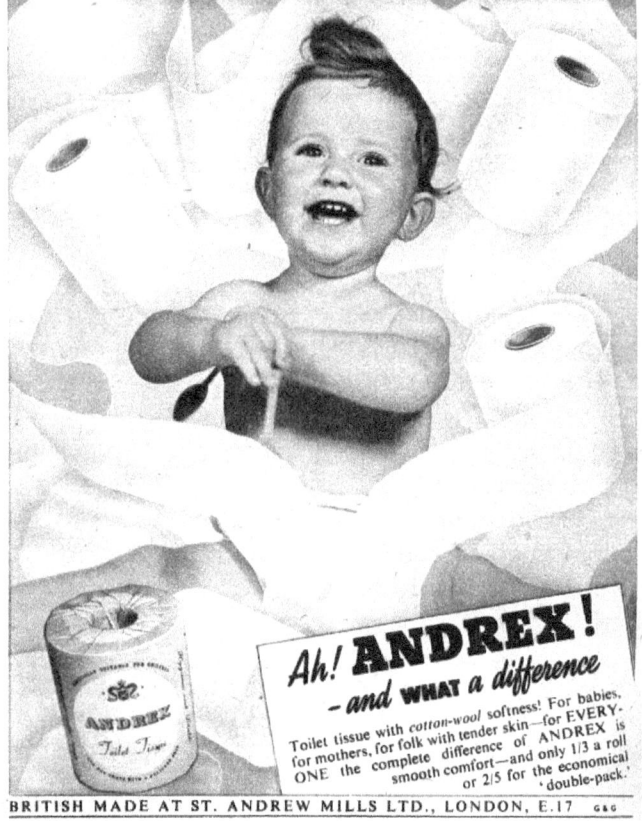

Figure 10: For Maximum benefit, make sure to start young

Paper not doing it for you? Try cardboard. The corrugated variety is better. You can even add flavouring or hot sauce if that's what floats your boat. It's all good as far as we're concerned.

The downside:

While this weight loss tip totally works, you can actually swap out all real food from your diet using this method - you may starve to death.

You also have to bear in mind that most paper products - toilet paper especially, are treated with bleach, which as you may or may not know, is really bad for you and kind of poisonous too. If it's the wrong kind of bleach which has been used and if there's enough of it left in your paper of choice, it can react with your stomach acid in a really bad way. Like, explosion bad.

Lastly, we've heard that consuming paper can do nasty things to your appendix. We don't actually know whether or not this is true, but you may want to give it a thought.

Meet my little friend

Death by malnutrition is a big problem throughout the developing world. It may not be that the kids are starving to death because they don't have enough to eat. It could be that they're just not eating the right things, or it could even be that the meagre nutrients they do consume are being sucked from their infant bodies by big nasty parasites.

Yes, that's right. Parasites which live in the gut and whose job it is to make sure that the nutrients from food don't get to where they're needed.

In the third world they may be parasites, but for the purpose of removing lard from your overly ample frame we're going to be looking at them as friends. Someone with whom you can work to ensure that you both get what you need. A symbiote if you will - the 'symbiote' gets fat, while you get thin like someone out a Stephen King novel. Everybody's happy.

Ideally, the parasite you want is a tapeworm. These are 'parasitic' flatworms of the phylum Platyhelminthes, and they are now your best friends.

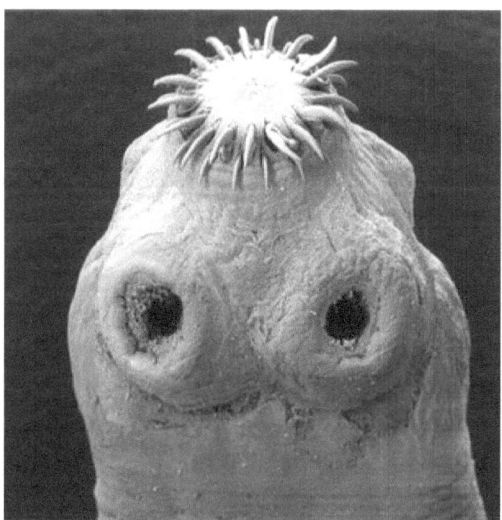

Figure 11: Say hello

Once installed in your gut, they will simply sit there growing larger, and larger as they absorb all of the goodness which floats by them. You need to do literally nothing else.

Finding a tapeworm you can live with and love is easy. The eggs can be bought as pills over the internet, however these can be expensive, difficult to swallow, and there is no guarantee they will latch on.

Luckily for you, tapeworms come in a variety of flavours which can affect humans, as they can be actually found in the muscles of their host animals.

For example, you can get Taenia saginata from beef, Taenia solium from pork, and Diphyllobothrium latum from fish. All of these are perfectly at home in the human gut, but as humans are not their natural host, most will not start burrowing through your flesh. So that's nice.

Unfortunately, you won't be able to catch a tapeworm from just any meat or reputable restaurant. You need to eat something of dubious provenance, severely undercooked, and with no record of the farm it was raised on. If you followed are advice in the 'Eat out and eat dirty' section, you may be lucky enough to already have a tapeworm living in you.

The downside:

Most people with a tapeworm won't show any symptoms outside of fabulous weight loss, and the fact that their faeces now move of their own accord.
Some people may also experience fatigue and weakness as the vitamins and nutrients they would normally absorb are sapped from their system by your new little symbiotic buddy.
Also, while we said that most tapeworms will not start burrowing through your flesh, this is not the case with pork tapeworms, which are perfectly at home in the human body and can make their way to your liver, eyes, heart, and brain. And when they get there, they can totally murder you.

We have also heard tales that a girl who was infected with a tapeworm was being taken up the poop chute by her boyfriend. When he withdrew, it was wrapped around his manly member. Vomit and terror ensued. However, we heard that on 4chan, so it probably isn't true. It might be though.

The Heisenberg Principle

We haven't seen the AMC TV series, Breaking bad. We've heard good things about it, but really, we watched the first couple of episodes, but couldn't really sympathise with the characters.

As far as we can tell, it's about a respected high school chemistry teacher who contracts cancer and starts his life anew as the best crystal meth chef and dealer in New Mexico. He gets rich and dies, leaving a trail of bodies in his wake.

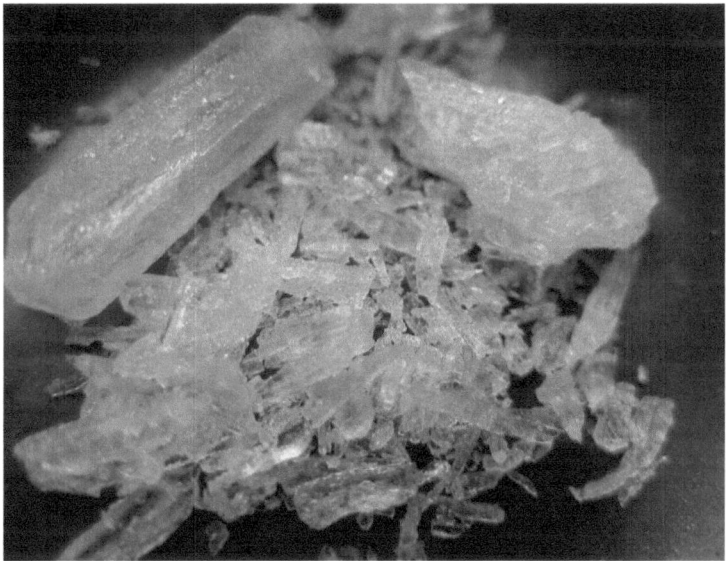

Figure 12: We were surprised to find out that crystal meth is not blue.

Crystal meth, or methamphetamine, is the nuclear option when it comes to weight loss. Once you pop, you can never stop. And you'll lose more than weight. Unless you start your habit when you're incredibly rich, you'll also lose every shred of dignity you've owned. And your teeth, your friends, probably your dog, too.

It's part of the amphetamine family we mentioned in 'Party like it's 1989,' but in reality, it's nothing like speed. Crystal meth is not something you can use occasionally for a night out, dancing.

As an amphetamine, it will have a stimulant effect, it will

accelerate your metabolism to an astronomical degree, and for the first few times you use it, you will feel fantastic and you will look slim.

People will want to have sex with you, and while you're on crystal meth, it will be the best sex you've ever had. We will reiterate: You will look and feel fabulous.

The downside:

It will not last. In an incredibly short time, the pleasure circuits of your brain will be burned out. There's a very severe high, followed by a severe comedown. As mentioned, it is very addictive, leaving you no option but to take more and more crystal.

Watch Breaking Bad, because that doesn't romanticise it at all.

But hey, you've got to to do what you've got to do. Right?

Combolicious

Some things in life go together beautifully. Cheese is a natural match for crackers; vodka complements Red Bull; quadruple salami is the perfect topping for a deep pan, stuffed crust 18 inch pizza.

Similarly, certain pieces of dieting advice can be taken together. Other pieces probably should not.

For instance caffeine and cigarettes are a match made in heaven. We've been up since six in the morning, and we've fuelled ourselves on a complete diet of nicotine and coffee, Not a single piece of solid food has passed our lips, and you know what? We've been working hard and we feel fucking fantastic, genuinely. Not even a little bit hungry. We could keep on going for hours - all night if necessary.

Granted, we've made our way through a bankrupting six packets of Marlboro red, but what were we going to spend that money on anyway.

The vodka trick works on every day of the week, and can be used to counteract the effects of the caffeine, albeit at potentially great personal cost, and a severely abbreviated lifespan if used long-term. So they work well together.

A example of a combination we would not recommend would be combining the advice from 'Snack Attack' with 'Say hello to my little friend.' you will end up getting no nutrition whatsoever, and you will end up in hospital quickly.

We do not think that crystal meth use is a good idea under any circumstances. However, it is extremely good as a weight loss drug, so really, we'd be negligent if we didn't mention it.

It's your life, so it's up to you in the end.

Afterword Haiku

We are not doctors.

This shit can fuck you up bad

But you will lose weight

ABOUT THE AUTHOR

Thomas Ap Dewi is a travel writer who has lived, worked and travelled in dozens of countries throughout the world. He usually writes travel guides, and what he doesn't know about far away places would fill several encyclopaedias.

He's a moderately clever chap, and some people think he's quite funny. Other people do not. Your own mileage may vary. While every effort has been made to ensure the accuracy of his books, some outright lies may have been included. But only when they're really easy to spot.